I0504215

TABLE OF CONTENTS

Chapter 1: Introduction to Mind Control

Our mind is a powerful tool that can either be our greatest ally or our worst enemy. It has the ability to control our thoughts, emotions, and behaviors, and ultimately influences our physical and mental health. Mind control refers to the ability to regulate and manage our thoughts, emotions, and behaviors in order to improve our overall well-being.

At its core, mind control involves the ability to recognize and control our thought patterns. Our thoughts can have a profound impact on our emotions, which in turn can affect our physical health. For example, chronic negative thoughts and stress can lead to a weakened immune system, high blood pressure, and even heart disease. On the other hand, positive thoughts and emotions can boost our immune system, improve our mood, and enhance our overall health.

Learning how to control our mind is essential for achieving a healthy and fulfilling life. By controlling our thoughts and emotions, we can reduce stress, anxiety, and depression. We can also improve our relationships, enhance our performance at work or school, and even overcome addictions and other destructive behaviors.

In this book, we will explore various techniques and strategies for mind control, including mindfulness meditation, yoga, exercise, diet, and mind-body techniques. We will also discuss how to overcome negative thoughts and anxieties, which can be major obstacles to achieving a healthy mind and body.

By learning how to control our mind, we can unlock our full potential and achieve a more fulfilling and satisfying life. Whether you are struggling with stress, weight gain, sickness, or negative thoughts, this book will provide you with the tools and knowledge you need to take control of your mind and improve your overall well-being.

The human mind is a complex and multifaceted entity that governs our thoughts, emotions, and behaviors. It is a source of immense power and can be our greatest asset, but it can also be our greatest hindrance if not properly managed. Mind control is the art of managing our thoughts, emotions, and behaviors to promote positive health outcomes and personal well-being.

The mind-body connection is well established in the scientific community, with many studies linking our thoughts and emotions to our physical health. Chronic stress, for example, has been shown to weaken the immune system, increase the risk of heart disease and stroke, and even lead to premature death. Conversely, positive emotions,

such as joy, love, and gratitude, have been linked to improved immune function, reduced inflammation, and improved cardiovascular health.

The concept of mind control can be understood through a few key concepts. The first is self-awareness, or the ability to observe and understand our own thoughts, emotions, and behaviors. By developing a greater sense of self-awareness, we can begin to recognize patterns in our thoughts and behaviors that may be contributing to negative health outcomes.

Another key concept in mind control is self-regulation, or the ability to manage our thoughts, emotions, and behaviors in a way that promotes positive health outcomes. This involves developing skills in stress management, emotion regulation, and impulse control.

The final key concept in mind control is self-transcendence, or the ability to move beyond our own personal concerns and connect with something greater than ourselves. This can involve developing a sense of purpose or meaning in life, engaging in acts of service or altruism, or connecting with nature or the divine.

These are all ways in which individuals can enhance their overall well-being and lead a more fulfilling life. Whether it's through pursuing one's passions and interests, giving back to others in meaningful ways, or finding solace and peace in the natural world or spiritual practices, there are many paths towards greater happiness and contentment. By cultivating a sense of purpose, empathy, and connection, individuals can build stronger relationships, improve their mental and physical health, and experience a deeper sense of joy and fulfillment in their daily lives.

There are many different techniques and practices that can be used to promote mind control and improve our overall well-being. These include:

1.Mindfulness meditation: This practice involves focusing your attention on the present moment and developing a non-judgmental awareness of your thoughts and emotions.
2.Yoga: This ancient practice combines physical postures, breathing techniques, and meditation to promote physical, mental, and emotional health.
3.Exercise: Regular exercise has been shown to improve mood, reduce stress, and improve physical health.
4.Diet: A healthy diet that includes plenty of fruits, vegetables, whole grains, and lean protein can provide the nutrients needed for optimal health and well-being.
5.Mind-body techniques: These techniques, such as hypnosis, guided imagery, and biofeedback, can help individuals to better regulate their thoughts, emotions, and behaviors.
6.Cognitive-behavioral therapy (CBT): This form of therapy helps individuals to identify and challenge negative thought patterns and behaviors that may be contributing to negative health outcomes.
By incorporating these techniques into our daily lives, we can develop greater control over our thoughts, emotions, and behaviors, and ultimately improve our overall well-being. Mind control is not about suppressing or denying our thoughts and emotions, but rather developing the skills and practices to manage them in a way that promotes positive health outcomes.

Chapter 2: Understanding Stress

Stress is a natural and inevitable part of life that affects everyone at some point. It can be defined as a physical, mental, or emotional response to a perceived challenge or demand, whether it's a major life event or a daily hassle. Stress can be helpful in motivating us to take action and solve problems, but when it becomes chronic or overwhelming, it can have negative impacts on our physical and mental health.
Types of Stress:
There are three main types of stress: acute stress, episodic acute stress, and chronic stress.
Acute stress is the most common type of stress and is usually caused by a specific event or situation, such as a job interview, a traffic jam, or an argument with a loved one. It's a normal and even necessary response that helps us to cope with challenges and take appropriate action. Acute stress can have positive effects, such as improving performance, enhancing focus and concentration, and boosting creativity.
Episodic acute stress is characterized by repeated episodes of acute stress, often caused by a pattern of negative thinking or behavior. People who experience this type of stress may feel like they are constantly in a state of crisis or chaos, and may exhibit symptoms such as anxiety, irritability, and even physical symptoms like headaches or stomach aches.

Chronic stress is long-term stress that can be caused by a variety of factors, including work, family, financial issues, or health problems. This type of stress can be particularly harmful to our physical and mental health and can lead to conditions such as depression, anxiety, heart disease, and obesity. Chronic stress can also have negative impacts on our cognitive function, including our ability to concentrate, make decisions, and remember things.

How Stress Affects the Body and Mind:
When we experience stress, the body's stress response is triggered, which involves the release of stress hormones like cortisol and adrenaline. These hormones prepare the body for "fight or flight" by increasing heart rate, blood pressure, and respiration. This response is designed to help us deal with immediate threats, but chronic stress can keep this response activated for prolonged periods of time, which can lead to a variety of negative effects on our physical and mental health. Chronic stress can weaken the immune system, making us more susceptible to illnesses and infections. It can also increase the risk of chronic diseases such as heart disease, stroke, and diabetes. Chronic stress can also contribute to mental health problems such as anxiety, depression, and burnout. It can also have negative impacts on our cognitive function, including our ability to concentrate, make decisions, and remember things.

Tamed Stress:

Fortunately, there are many strategies that can be used to tame stress and promote a healthy response to stress. These include:

1.Exercise: Regular exercise can help to reduce stress and improve mood. Exercise can also improve sleep quality, boost energy levels, and reduce the risk of chronic

diseases.
2.Mindfulness meditation: This practice involves focusing your attention on the present moment and developing a non-judgmental awareness of your thoughts and emotions. Mindfulness meditation can help to reduce stress, improve mood, and enhance cognitive function.

3.Relaxation techniques: These techniques, such as deep breathing exercises or progressive muscle relaxation, can help to reduce muscle tension and
promote relaxation. Relaxation techniques can also improve sleep quality and reduce symptoms of anxiety and depression.

4.Social support: Having a strong social support system can help to buffer the negative effects of stress and provide emotional support during challenging times. Social support can come from friends, family, coworkers, or support groups.
5.Time management: Learning to manage your time effectively can help to reduce stress and prevent feeling overwhelmed. This can involve setting priorities, delegating tasks, and avoiding procrastination.

By incorporating these strategies into your daily life, you can develop greater resilience to stress and improve your overall well-being. It's important to remember that managing stress is not about eliminating stress altogether, but rather finding healthy ways to cope with stress and minimize its negative effects.

It's also important to recognize when stress has become too much to handle on your own and to seek professional help if needed. This can include therapy, counseling, or medication, depending on the individual's needs and situation.

In conclusion, understanding stress is the first step in learning to manage it effectively. By recognizing

the different types of stress and how it affects our body and mind, we can begin to develop healthy coping strategies that promote resilience and well-being. It's never too late to start taking steps to manage stress and improve our quality of life.

Chapter 3: Causes of Stress

Stress is a natural and normal part of life, and it can be caused by a variety of factors. Some sources of stress are minor and short-lived, while others can be more significant and long-term. It's important to identify the causes of stress in your life so that you can learn to manage them effectively and reduce their impact on your physical and mental health. In this chapter, we will explore some common causes of stress.

Work-related Stress:

Work-related stress is a common source of stress for many people. It can be caused by a variety of factors, such as job demands, lack of control or autonomy, conflict with coworkers or supervisors, or work-life balance issues. Job demands can include workload, time pressure, and conflicting priorities. Lack of control or autonomy can be caused by micromanagement or feeling like your ideas and opinions are not valued. Conflict with coworkers or supervisors can cause tension and stress in the workplace. Work-life balance issues can result from long work hours, lack of flexibility, or feeling like work is taking over your personal life.

Prolonged exposure to work-related stress can lead to physical and mental health problems such as headaches, stomach problems, high blood pressure, depression, and anxiety. Therefore, it is important to learn to manage work-related stress to avoid long-term negative effects on your well-being.

Relationship Stress:

Relationships can be a source of stress, whether it's with a romantic partner, family member, friend, or coworker. Relationship stress can be caused by a variety of factors, such as communication problems, disagreements, conflicts, or changes in the relationship. Communication problems can occur when there is a lack of understanding or misinterpretation of messages. Disagreements and conflicts can arise from differences in opinions, values, or goals. Changes in the relationship, such as a break-up, divorce, or loss of a loved one, can also be a significant source of stress. Just as work related stress prolonged exposure to relationship stress can lead to physical and mental health problems such as headaches, insomnia, anxiety,
and depression. Therefore, it is important to learn effective communication skills and conflict resolution techniques to manage relationship stress.

Financial Stress:

Financial stress is a common source of stress for many people. It can be caused by a variety of factors, such as debt, job loss, unexpected expenses, or living beyond your means. Debt can cause stress by creating a sense of financial insecurity and pressure to make payments. Job loss can cause stress by creating uncertainty about the future and the ability to make ends meet. Unexpected expenses, such as car repairs or medical bills, can create financial strain. Living beyond your means, such as overspending or not saving enough, can create long-term financial stress.

Trauma and Grief:

Trauma and grief can be significant sources of stress. Trauma can be caused by experiencing or witnessing a traumatic event, such as a natural disaster, violence, or abuse. Grief can be caused by the loss of a loved one or a significant life change, such as a divorce or job loss. Trauma and grief can cause stress by creating feelings of sadness, anger, and anxiety. These emotions can be difficult to manage and can interfere with daily life. Once again, prolonged exposure to trauma and grief can lead to physical and mental health problems such as post-traumatic stress disorder (PTSD), depression, and anxiety. Therefore, it is important to seek professional help, such as therapy or counseling, to manage trauma and grief-related stress.

Managing Stress:

Identifying the sources of stress in your life is the first step in managing stress. Once you have identified the sources of stress, you can develop strategies to manage them effectively. This may include developing healthy coping mechanisms, such as exercise, mindfulness, or relaxation techniques. It may also involve making changes to your lifestyle or seeking professional help, such as therapy or counseling.
In conclusion, stress can be caused by a variety of factors, including work-related stress, relationship stress, financial stress, and trauma and grief. Identifying the sources of stress in your life is the first step in managing stress effectively. By developing healthy coping strategies and seeking professional help when needed, you can reduce the impact of stress on your physical and mental health.

Chapter 4: The Physiology of Stress

The stress response system is a complex physiological process that prepares the body to deal with perceived threats or challenges. The system involves the hypothalamus, the pituitary gland, and the adrenal glands, collectively known as the HPA axis. When a person experiences stress, the hypothalamus releases a hormone called corticotropin-releasing hormone (CRH), which triggers the pituitary gland to release adrenocorticotropic hormone (ACTH). ACTH then stimulates the adrenal glands to produce cortisol and other stress hormones.

The effects of stress hormones on the body are numerous and can have both short-term and long-term consequences. In the short term, cortisol and other stress hormones increase heart rate and blood pressure, dilate air passages to improve breathing, and increase blood sugar levels to provide energy to the muscles. These effects help the body to cope with the perceived threat or challenge.

However, chronic or long-term stress can have negative effects on the body. Prolonged exposure to cortisol and other stress hormones can lead to a weakened immune system, increased risk of infection, and impaired cognitive function. Chronic stress can also contribute to the development of cardiovascular disease, metabolic disorders, and other health problems.

Additionally, chronic stress can affect the brain and the nervous system. It can lead to structural and functional changes in the brain, including shrinkage of the prefrontal cortex and enlargement of the amygdala, which can contribute to anxiety and depression. Chronic stress can also affect neurotransmitter systems in the brain, including the dopamine and serotonin systems, which can further contribute to mood disorders.

In summary, while the stress response system is an important mechanism for helping the body cope with perceived threats or challenges, chronic stress can have negative effects on the body and the brain. It is important to manage stress through relaxation techniques, exercise, and other stress-reducing strategies to promote overall health and well-being.

One way chronic stress can affect the body is by contributing to the development of cardiovascular

disease. Long-term exposure to stress hormones can lead to increased blood pressure, inflammation, and changes in the way blood vessels function, all of which can contribute to the development of atherosclerosis and other cardiovascular problems. Chronic stress has also been linked to an increased risk of heart attack, stroke, and other cardiovascular events.

Chronic stress can also affect the immune system, which can increase the risk of infections and other health problems. Prolonged exposure to cortisol and other stress hormones can suppress the immune system, making it more difficult for the body to fight off infections and diseases. Chronic stress has been linked to an increased risk of infections, autoimmune disorders, and even cancer. In addition to physical health problems, chronic stress can also affect mental health. Chronic stress has been linked to an increased risk of anxiety and depression, as well as other mood disorders. Prolonged exposure to stress hormones can lead to changes in the way the brain functions, including changes in the levels of neurotransmitters like serotonin and dopamine, which can contribute to mood disorders. Overall, chronic stress can have negative effects on the body and the brain. It is important to manage stress through relaxation techniques, exercise, and other stress-reducing strategies to promote overall health and well-being.

Seeking professional help if necessary, such as through therapy or medication, can also be beneficial in managing chronic stress and its effects. You can simply take a chill pill
(Pun intended) which can be very effective as long as it doesn't become abusive.There are various organic strategies (no pills) that individuals can use to manage stress and reduce its negative effects. One effective strategy is exercise, which can help reduce stress levels and improve overall physical and mental health. Exercise can also stimulate the release of endorphins, which are natural mood-boosters.

Another strategy is practicing relaxation techniques, such as deep breathing, meditation, or yoga. These techniques can help reduce stress levels and promote relaxation, which can have numerous benefits for both the body and mind. Additionally, engaging in activities that bring joy and pleasure, such as hobbies or spending time with loved ones, can help reduce stress levels and promote overall well-being.

For some individuals, seeking professional help may be necessary to manage chronic stress and its
effects. This can include therapy, medication, or a combination of both. Therapy can help individuals develop coping skills and strategies to manage stress more effectively, while medication can help alleviate symptoms of anxiety or depression.

In conclusion, the stress response system is an important physiological process that prepares the body to deal with perceived threats or challenges. However, chronic stress can have negative effects on the body and the brain, leading to a range of health problems. It is important to manage stress through various strategies, such as exercise, relaxation techniques, and seeking professional help when necessary, to promote overall health and well-being.

Chapter 5: Mindful Meditation

Mindful meditation (a commonly used term that actually works) is a form of meditation that involves paying attention to the present moment with curiosity and non-judgmental awareness. It is a technique that has been used for centuries in various cultures and is now becoming more widely recognized as a powerful tool for reducing stress and improving overall well-being.

Definition of Mindful Meditation:

Mindful meditation involves intentionally focusing one's attention on the present moment, without judgment or distraction. This involves paying attention to physical sensations, thoughts, and emotions, and observing them without becoming attached to them or reacting to them.

The practice of mindfulness meditation encourages individuals to become more aware of their own mental and emotional processes, and to develop a more compassionate and accepting attitude towards themselves and others. This can help individuals to cultivate greater inner peace, clarity of mind, and a greater sense of overall well-being.

The practice of mindfulness meditation encourages individuals to become more aware of their own mental and emotional processes, and to develop a more compassionate and accepting attitude towards themselves and others. This can help individuals to cultivate greater inner peace, clarity of mind, and a greater sense of overall well-being.

How Mindfulness Can Reduce Stress

Research has shown that mindfulness meditation can be an effective tool for reducing stress and its negative effects on the body and mind. The practice of mindfulness can help individuals to reduce anxiety, depression, and other mood disorders, and can also improve sleep quality and overall physical health.

One of the key ways that mindful meditation can reduce stress is by helping individuals to become more aware of their own thoughts and emotions, and to develop a more positive and accepting attitude towards them. By cultivating greater self-awareness and self-compassion, individuals can become better equipped to cope with stressful situations and to manage their emotional responses to them.

Mindful meditation can also help individuals to develop a greater sense of present-moment awareness, which can help to reduce feelings of overwhelm and anxiety. By focusing on the present moment, individuals can reduce their tendency to ruminate on past or future events, which can contribute to feelings of stress and anxiety.

Techniques for Practicing Mindful Meditation

There are various techniques that individuals can use to practice mindfulness meditation. Some of these techniques include:

1.Focused breathing - this involves focusing one's attention on the sensations of the breath, such as the movement of the chest or the feeling of air passing through the nostrils.
2.Body scan - this involves paying attention to different parts of the body, starting at the toes and working up to the top of the head, and observing any physical sensations without judgment.
3.Mindful movement - this involves performing physical movements, such as yoga or tai chi, while focusing one's attention on the sensations of the body and breath.
4.Loving-kindness meditation - this involves directing positive thoughts and feelings towards oneself and others, with the intention of cultivating greater compassion and kindness.
It is important to note that mindfulness meditation is not a quick fix for stress or other mental health problems. It is a practice that requires ongoing commitment and patience, and may take time to develop.

Additionally, research has shown that regular mindfulness meditation practice can lead to structural and functional changes in the brain, which may contribute to its positive effects on mental health. Specifically, regular practice has been associated with increased activity in the prefrontal cortex, a part of the brain that is involved in decision-making, attention, and emotional regulation.

Furthermore, mindfulness meditation has been found to be helpful for individuals with a wide range of mental health conditions, including anxiety disorders, depression, and post-traumatic stress disorder (PTSD). It has also been found to be helpful in managing chronic pain and improving immune system functioning.

Here are some tips for individuals who are interested in practicing mindfulness meditation:

Set aside time each day to practice mindfulness meditation, even if it's just a few minutes. Consistency is key to experiencing the benefits of the practice.

Find a quiet and comfortable place to meditate where you won't be interrupted.

Start with shorter periods of meditation and gradually increase the length of your sessions as you become more comfortable with the practice.

Focus on your breath and try to bring your attention back to your breath whenever your mind begins to wander.

Practice self-compassion and avoid judging yourself if you find it difficult to focus or if you experience uncomfortable thoughts or emotions.

In summary, mindfulness meditation is a powerful tool for reducing stress and improving overall well-being. Its benefits extend beyond stress reduction, including improvements in mental health, physical health, and brain functioning.

By incorporating mindfulness meditation into one's daily routine, individuals can develop greater resilience and coping skills, and improve their overall quality of life.

In summary, mindfulness meditation is a powerful tool for reducing stress and improving overall well-being. The practice involves intentionally focusing one's attention on the present moment, without judgment or distraction, and can help individuals to cultivate greater self-awareness, self-compassion, and present-moment awareness.

By incorporating mindfulness meditation into one's daily routine, individuals can develop greater resilience and coping skills, and improve their overall mental and physical health.

Chapter 6: Yoga and Stress Reduction

Yoga is an ancient practice that has been around for over 5,000 years. It originated in India and has since spread all over the world. Yoga is a combination of physical postures, breathing techniques, and meditation. The practice of yoga has been found to be an effective tool for stress reduction and improving overall well-being.

Definition of Yoga

Yoga is a physical, mental, and spiritual practice that originated in India. It involves physical postures, breathing techniques, and meditation. The practice of yoga aims to unite the mind, body, and spirit, and to promote overall health and well-being.

The Benefits of Yoga for Stress Reduction

Yoga has been found to be an effective tool for reducing stress and its negative effects on the body and mind. The practice of yoga can help to reduce anxiety, depression, and other mood disorders, and can also improve sleep quality and overall physical health.

One of the key ways that yoga can reduce stress is by promoting relaxation and reducing muscle tension.

The physical postures, or asanas, of yoga are designed to stretch and strengthen the body, which can help to release tension and promote relaxation. The breathing techniques, or pranayama, of yoga can also help to reduce stress by promoting relaxation and calming the mind.

In addition to its physical benefits, the practice of yoga can also help individuals to develop greater self-awareness and self-compassion. This can help to reduce feelings of overwhelm and anxiety, and can also promote greater emotional regulation and resilience.

Types of Yoga that are Best for Stress Reduction

There are many different types of yoga, each with their own unique benefits and focus. When it comes to stress reduction, some types of yoga are more beneficial than others. Here are some of the types of yoga that are best for stress reduction:

1.Hatha Yoga - This is a gentle and slow-paced form of yoga that is focused on physical postures and breathing techniques. It is a great option for beginners and those who are looking for a more gentle form of yoga.

2.Restorative Yoga - This is a very gentle and relaxing form of yoga that is focused on relaxation and rest. It involves using props, such as blankets and bolsters, to support the body in passive postures that are held for longer periods of time.

3.Yin Yoga - This is a slow-paced form of yoga that is focused on stretching and holding postures for longer periods of time. It is a great option for those who are looking for a more meditative form of yoga.

4.Vinyasa Yoga - This is a more dynamic form of yoga that involves flowing from one posture to another in a sequence. It is a great option for those who are looking for a more active form of yoga.

Tips for Practicing Yoga for Stress Reduction

If you are interested in incorporating yoga into your routine to reduce stress, here are some tips to get started:

1.Start with a beginner's class - If you are new to yoga, it's a good idea to start with a beginner's class. This will allow you to learn the basics and develop good alignment and breathing techniques.

2.Focus on your breath - Breathing is a key part of yoga and can help to promote relaxation and reduce stress. Focus on your breath during your practice, and try to synchronize your breath with your movements.

3.Use props - Props, such as blocks, straps, and blankets, can help to support your body during postures and make them more accessible. Don't be afraid to use props if you need them.

4.Don't push yourself too hard - It's important to listen to your body and not push yourself too hard. Yoga is not a competitive sport, and it's important to honor your body's limitations.

5.Practice regularly - Consistency is key when it comes to yoga. Aim to practice yoga regularly, even if it's just for a few minutes each day. Over time, you will begin to notice the benefits of your practice.

In conclusion, yoga is a powerful tool for reducing stress and improving overall well-being. The physical postures, breathing techniques, and meditation of yoga can help individuals to reduce muscle tension, promote relaxation, and develop greater self-awareness and self-compassion.

When it comes to stress reduction, there are many different types of yoga to choose from, each with their own unique benefits and focus.

By incorporating yoga into one's daily routine, individuals can develop greater resilience and coping skills, and improve their overall mental and physical health.

Chapter 7: Exercise and Stress Reduction

Exercise is well-known for its physical benefits, but did you know that it can also be an effective way to reduce stress? Exercise is a natural stress reliever that can help to improve mood, reduce muscle tension, and promote relaxation. In this chapter, we will explore the benefits of exercise for stress reduction, the types of exercise that are best for stress reduction, and how much exercise is needed to reduce stress.

The Benefits of Exercise for Stress Reduction

Exercise can help to reduce stress in a number of ways. First, it promotes the release of endorphins, which are natural mood boosters that can help to reduce feelings of anxiety and depression. Second, exercise can help to reduce muscle tension, which is a common physical symptom of stress. By engaging in physical activity, you can help to release pent-up tension and feel more relaxed. Third, exercise can promote better sleep, which is essential for reducing stress levels. Finally, exercise can help to boost self-confidence and self-esteem, which can help to reduce feelings of stress and anxiety.

Types of Exercise that are Best for Stress Reduction

While any type of exercise can be beneficial for reducing stress, some types of exercise are better than others. The best types of exercise for stress reduction are those that involve rhythmic, repetitive movements and focus on breath control. These types of exercises include:

Aerobic exercise - Aerobic exercise, such as running, cycling, or swimming, can help to reduce stress levels by promoting the release of endorphins and reducing muscle tension.
Yoga - Yoga combines physical postures with breathing techniques and meditation to promote relaxation and reduce stress.
Tai Chi - Tai Chi is a low-impact form of exercise that combines gentle movements with deep breathing to promote relaxation and reduce stress.
Pilates - Pilates is a form of exercise that focuses on core strength, flexibility, and breath control, making it an effective way to reduce stress levels.
How Much Exercise is Needed to Reduce Stress?

The amount of exercise needed to reduce stress varies depending on individual needs and preferences. However, research suggests that engaging in regular exercise for at least 30 minutes a day, five days a week, can help to reduce stress levels.

It's important to note that the benefits of exercise for stress reduction are cumulative, so even small amounts of exercise can help to reduce stress levels over time.

Tips for Incorporating Exercise into Your Routine for Stress Reduction

If you are interested in incorporating exercise into your routine to reduce stress, here are some tips to get started:

Choose activities you enjoy - Exercise doesn't have to be a chore. Choose activities that you enjoy, whether it's dancing, swimming, or hiking. This will make it more likely that you stick with your exercise routine over the long term.
Make it a part of your routine - Consistency is key when it comes to exercise. Make it a part of your daily routine, whether it's going for a walk after dinner or hitting the gym before work.
Start slowly - If you are new to exercise, it's important to start slowly and gradually build up your endurance. This will help to prevent injury and make it more likely that you stick with your exercise routine.
Focus on your breath - As we mentioned earlier, breathing is an important component of stress reduction. Focus on your breath during your workouts, and try to synchronize your breath with your movements.

Find a workout buddy - Exercising with a friend or family member can make it more enjoyable and provide additional motivation to stick with your routine.

In conclusion, exercise is a powerful tool for reducing stress and improving overall well-being. Its physical and psychological benefits can help individuals to reduce muscle tension, promote relaxation, and improve their overall mental and physical health.

By incorporating exercise into one's daily routine and engaging in activities that promote relaxation and breath control, individuals can develop greater resilience and coping skills, and reduce the negative impact of stress on their lives.

Any sort of voluntary physical activity is a natural stress reliever that can help to improve mood.

By choosing activities that you enjoy, making exercise a mandatory part of your life (suggested), starting slowly, focusing on your breath, and finding a workout buddy, you can develop greater resilience and coping skills, and improve your overall mental and physical health.

Chapter 8: Diet and Stress Reduction

Diet plays a crucial role in reducing stress because what we eat can impact our mood and overall well-being. Certain foods can help reduce stress, while others can actually increase it.

Let's start by discussing the effects of diet on stress. Our bodies need a variety of nutrients to function correctly. When we eat a healthy and balanced diet, we provide our bodies with the necessary nutrients to manage stress effectively.

For example, a diet rich in whole grains, fruits, and vegetables provides our bodies with essential vitamins and minerals, including B vitamins, magnesium, and vitamin C, which are important in reducing stress levels.

On the other hand, a poor diet can increase stress levels. Consuming high amounts of refined sugar, caffeine, and processed foods can lead to fluctuations in blood sugar levels and cause stress and anxiety. These types of foods can also affect our sleep patterns and make us more susceptible to stress.

So, what are the foods that can reduce stress levels? Here are some examples:

1.Dark chocolate: Dark chocolate is rich in flavonoids, which can reduce stress levels and improve mood.
2.Fatty fish: Fatty fish, such as salmon and tuna, are high in omega-3 fatty acids, which can help reduce inflammation and lower stress levels.
3.Nuts: Nuts, such as almonds and walnuts, are high in magnesium, which can reduce stress levels and improve sleep quality.
4.Fruits and vegetables: Fruits and vegetables are rich in antioxidants, vitamins, and minerals, which can help reduce stress levels and improve overall health.
5.Herbal teas: Certain herbal teas, such as chamomile and lavender tea, can have a calming effect and reduce stress levels.

Now, what are the foods that can increase stress levels? Here are some examples:

1.Refined sugar: Refined sugar can cause a spike in blood sugar levels, leading to feelings of anxiety and stress.
2.Caffeine: Caffeine can increase heart rate and blood pressure, leading to feelings of anxiety and stress.
3.Processed foods: Processed foods are often high in sodium and can cause dehydration, which can increase stress levels.
4.Alcohol: While alcohol may initially have a relaxing effect, it can also disrupt sleep patterns and increase stress levels.

We should always remember that our relationship with food will surely impact our stress levels one way or the other. Stress can cause us to turn to comfort foods or indulge in emotional eating, leading to unhealthy eating patterns. In contrast, a healthy relationship with food can promote healthy eating habits and reduce stress levels.

Here are some tips for promoting a healthy relationship with food and reducing stress levels:

1.Practice mindful eating: Mindful eating involves paying attention to the taste, texture, and smell of our food, as well as our hunger and fullness cues. This practice can help us develop a healthier relationship with food and reduce stress levels.
2.Avoid restrictive diets: Restrictive diets can lead to feelings of deprivation and increase stress levels. Instead, focus on a balanced and varied diet that includes a variety of foods.
3.Plan meals ahead of time: Planning meals ahead of time can reduce stress and make it easier to make healthy choices.
4.Avoid emotional eating: Emotional eating involves using food to cope with emotions, such as stress or sadness. Instead, try other coping mechanisms, such as exercise or meditation.
5.Seek support: If you struggle with a healthy relationship with food, seek support from a therapist, registered dietitian, or other healthcare professionals. Here are five healthy and tasty recipes that can help reduce stress:

1.Grilled salmon with avocado salsa: Salmon is a great source of omega-3 fatty acids, which can help reduce inflammation and lower stress levels. Avocado is also a great source of healthy fats and fiber. To make this dish, grill a salmon fillet and top it with a salsa made from avocado, tomato, onion, and lime juice.

2.Quinoa salad with roasted vegetables: Quinoa is a great source of protein and fiber, which can help keep you full and reduce stress levels. Roasted vegetables, such as sweet potatoes, broccoli, and red peppers, are a great source of vitamins and minerals.
To make this dish, cook quinoa according to package instructions and toss it with roasted vegetables and a dressing made from olive oil, lemon juice, and herbs.

3.Turkey and sweet potato chili: Turkey is a lean source of protein, and sweet potatoes are high in fiber and vitamins.

Chili can also be a great source of antioxidants from spices like chili powder and cumin. To make this dish, brown ground turkey and add chopped onions, garlic, diced tomatoes, and sweet potatoes. Season with chili powder, cumin, salt, and pepper, and let it simmer until the sweet potatoes are tender.

4.Berry and yogurt smoothie: Berries are high in antioxidants and can help reduce inflammation, while yogurt is a great source of probiotics and protein. To make this smoothie, blend frozen berries, plain Greek yogurt, almond milk, and honey until smooth.

5.Dark chocolate and almond bark: Dark chocolate contains flavonoids, which can help reduce stress levels and improve mood. Almonds are also a great source of healthy fats and protein.

To make this treat, melt dark chocolate and stir in chopped almonds. Spread the mixture on a baking sheet and let it cool in the refrigerator until firm. These recipes are all nutritious, delicious, and perfect with a healthy and satisfying taste . Enjoy!

I know what your thinking, What happen to the salads?"

Here are three healthy and delicious salad recipes:

1.Grilled chicken and strawberry salad: This salad is a perfect combination of sweet and savory flavors and is loaded with nutrients. To make this salad, start by grilling chicken breasts and slicing them into strips.

In a large bowl, mix together fresh spinach, sliced strawberries, sliced almonds, crumbled feta cheese, and grilled chicken. Drizzle with a balsamic vinaigrette made with olive oil, balsamic vinegar, honey, and Dijon mustard.

2.Mediterranean quinoa salad: This salad is loaded with fiber, protein, and healthy fats and is perfect for a light and refreshing meal. Cook quinoa according to package instructions and let it cool. In a large bowl, mix together the cooked quinoa, chopped cherry tomatoes, diced cucumber, crumbled feta cheese, sliced Kalamata olives, and chopped fresh parsley. Drizzle with a lemon and olive oil dressing.

3.Kale Caesar salad: This salad is a healthy twist on a classic Caesar salad, with added nutrients from kale and quinoa. Start by cooking quinoa according to package instructions and let it cool. In a large bowl, mix together chopped kale, cooked quinoa, sliced cherry tomatoes, and sliced red onion. Toss with a homemade Caesar dressing made with Greek yogurt, Dijon mustard, garlic, lemon juice, and Parmesan cheese.

These recipes are all delicious and packed with nutrients that can help reduce stress levels. Remember to enjoy them in moderation and as part of a balanced and varied diet.

Chapter 9: Mentally Understanding Weight Gain

Weight gain is a common issue that affects many people worldwide. It is the gradual increase in body weight over time, typically resulting from an imbalance between the number of calories consumed and the number of calories burned. While some weight gain can be healthy, excessive weight gain can lead to various health issues, such as obesity, diabetes, heart disease, and mental health problems.

Causes of Weight Gain:
There are several factors that can contribute to weight gain, including:
1.Poor diet: Eating a diet high in calories, processed foods, and added sugars can contribute to weight gain.
2.Lack of physical activity: A sedentary lifestyle with little to no exercise can contribute to weight gain.
3.Genetics: Some people may be more prone to weight gain due to their genes.
4.Medical conditions: Certain medical conditions, such as hypothyroidism and Cushing's syndrome, can lead to weight gain.
5.Medications: Some medications, such as antidepressants and corticosteroids, can cause weight gain.
How Weight Gain Affects the Body and Mind:
Weight gain can have several negative effects on the body and mind, including:

1.Increased risk of chronic diseases: Excessive weight gain can increase the risk of chronic diseases, such as diabetes, heart disease, and cancer.

2.Poor mental health: Weight gain can also affect mental health, leading to issues such as depression, anxiety, and low self-esteem.

3.Joint pain: The excess weight can put pressure on the joints, leading to joint pain and inflammation.

4.Sleep apnea: Weight gain can contribute to sleep apnea, a condition in which breathing repeatedly stops and starts during sleep.

5.Reduced mobility: Excessive weight gain can reduce mobility and make it difficult to perform daily activities.

Ways to Manage Weight Gain:

1.Healthy diet: A healthy diet that includes a variety of fruits, vegetables, lean protein, and whole grains can help manage weight gain.

2.Regular exercise: Regular exercise can help burn calories and improve overall health.

3.Mindful eating: Practicing mindful eating by paying attention to hunger and fullness cues and eating slowly can help prevent overeating.

4.Managing stress: Stress can contribute to weight gain, so managing stress through relaxation techniques such as meditation, yoga, and deep breathing can be helpful.

5.Adequate sleep: Getting enough sleep can help manage weight gain, as sleep deprivation can lead to hormonal imbalances that can contribute to weight gain.

Tips for Healthy Weight Management:
Here are some additional tips to help manage weight gain in a healthy way: if you have a weight problem you should always keep that in MIND.

1.Set realistic goals: Setting realistic goals for weight loss or weight management can help you stay motivated and on track.

2.Keep a food journal: Keeping a food journal can help you become more aware of your eating habits and make healthier choices.

3.Drink plenty of water: Drinking plenty of water can help reduce hunger and prevent overeating.

4.Limit processed foods and added sugars: Processed foods and added sugars can contribute to weight gain, so it's important to limit their consumption.

5.Find a support system: Finding a support system, such as a friend or family member, can help you stay motivated and accountable.

6.Avoid fad diets: Fad diets that promise quick weight loss are often unhealthy and unsustainable, so it's best to avoid them.

7.Get professional help: If you're struggling with weight gain or have an underlying medical condition, it's important to seek professional help from a healthcare provider or registered dietitian.

By incorporating these tips and adopting healthy habits, we can manage weight gain in a healthy and sustainable way, improving our overall health and wellbeing by believing in our MINDS that we can.

Chapter 10: The psychology behind the Physiology of Weight Gain

It is important to understand that weight gain and obesity are complex conditions that cannot be solely attributed to individual behavior or personal choices. Mental health issues such as depression, anxiety, and stress can contribute to overeating or lack of physical activity, but these conditions do not equate to a mental deficiency.

The human body stores and uses energy in a complex process involving multiple organs and hormones. When we consume food, the body breaks it down into glucose, which is used as the primary source of energy for the cells. Any excess glucose is stored in the liver and muscles as glycogen, and when those stores are full, the excess is converted into fat and stored in adipose tissue.

Insulin is a hormone produced by the pancreas that plays a critical role in regulating glucose levels in the body. When glucose levels rise in the bloodstream, insulin is released to signal cells to take up glucose and use it for energy or store it for later use. Insulin also inhibits the breakdown of fat in adipose tissue, promoting the storage of fat in the body. Thus, high levels of insulin can contribute to weight gain.

Stress hormones, such as cortisol and adrenaline, are released by the body in response to stress.

These hormones trigger the release of glucose into the bloodstream, providing energy to deal with the stressful situation.

However, chronic stress can lead to consistently elevated levels of these hormones, which can promote the storage of fat in the body, especially around the abdomen.

In addition, stress can lead to emotional eating and the consumption of high-calorie, high-fat foods, further contributing to weight gain.

Mental coping strategies can help reduce the negative effects of stress on weight gain.

These strategies may include relaxation techniques, such as deep breathing or meditation, exercise, talking to a trusted friend or therapist, or engaging in a favorite hobby or activity.

Developing healthy coping mechanisms can help reduce stress and promote overall health and well-being.

Chapter 11: Mindful Eating

Mindful eating is a practice of paying attention to the food we eat, the sensations in our body, and our thoughts and emotions related to eating. It involves being fully present and engaged in the experience of eating, without distractions or judgments.

Mindful eating can help prevent weight gain by promoting a healthier relationship with food and reducing overeating.

When we eat mindfully, we pay attention to our body's hunger and fullness signals, which can help prevent overeating. We also become more aware of our food choices and the impact they have on our bodies, which can lead to healthier eating habits.

Mindful eating can also reduce stress and emotional eating by helping us tune in to our emotions and choose healthier coping mechanisms.

Here are some techniques for practicing mindful eating:

1.Slow down: Eat slowly and take the time to savor each bite. This allows your body to register feelings of fullness, reducing the likelihood of overeating.

2."your meal to express gratitude for the food and the people who prepared it. This can help you cultivate a positive relationship with food.

Our minds play a critical role in controlling what we eat. Our food choices are influenced by a complex interplay of biological, psychological, and social factors. The way we think and feel about food can impact our food choices, eating habits, and ultimately, our health.

Here are some ways our minds control what we eat:

1.Cravings and Food Preferences: Our minds can create cravings for specific types of food, such as salty or sweet foods. Our food preferences can also be influenced by factors such as our culture, family traditions, and personal experiences.

2.Emotional Eating: Our emotions can have a significant impact on our food choices. When we are stressed, anxious, or bored, we may turn to food as a way of coping with these emotions.

3.Habitual Eating: Our minds can create habits around eating, such as always reaching for a snack when watching TV or eating at a certain time of day.

4.Social Influence: Our minds can be influenced by our social environment, such as eating habits of our family or friends, and the availability and marketing of food.

41

5.Cognitive Processes: Our cognitive processes, such as attention and memory, can influence our food choices. For example, paying attention to nutrition labels can influence our food choices, and memories of positive food experiences can lead us to choose certain foods again in the future.

Additionally, our minds also control the quantity of food we eat. Research has shown that portion sizes play a significant role in overeating and weight gain.

Our minds can be influenced by the visual cues of portion sizes, such as the size of the plate or container, and we may end up eating more than we need to.

On the other hand, by practicing mindfulness and paying attention to our body's hunger and fullness signals, we can learn to control our portion sizes and eat until we are satisfied rather than overeating.

Another way our minds control what we eat is through our decision-making processes.When faced with food choices, our minds can evaluate the options based on factors such as taste, convenience, healthiness, and cost. By becoming more aware of these factors and making conscious decisions about what we eat, we can choose healthier options that align with our goals and values.

Finally, our minds can also control our eating behaviors through our self-talk and beliefs.

For example, negative self-talk and beliefs, such as "I have no willpower" or "I always overeat," can lead to a self-fulfilling prophecy and sabotage our efforts to make healthier choices.

By cultivating positive self-talk and beliefs, such as "I am capable of making healthy choices" or "I listen to my body's signals," we can empower ourselves to make positive changes in our eating habits.

In conclusion, our minds play a critical role in controlling what we eat. Factors such as cravings, emotional eating, habits, social influence, and cognitive processes can all impact our food choices and eating habits.

By practicing mindful eating and becoming more aware of these factors, we can take control of our eating habits and make healthier choices.

Chapter 12: Understanding How Sickness Affects The Body And Mind.

Definition of Sickness:
Sickness refers to a state of physical or mental illness or discomfort that affects the normal functioning of the body or mind. It can be caused by a variety of factors such as infections, injuries, chronic conditions, genetic predispositions, environmental factors, and lifestyle choices.
Causes of Sickness:
The causes of sickness can vary greatly and may include:
1.Infectious agents such as viruses, bacteria, fungi, and parasites.
2.Genetic predispositions or inherited disorders that affect the normal functioning of the body.
3.Environmental factors such as exposure to toxins, pollution, or radiation.
4.Lifestyle choices such as poor diet, lack of exercise, and smoking.
5.Chronic conditions such as diabetes, hypertension, and heart disease.
6.Injuries such as fractures, cuts, and burns.
7.Psychological factors such as stress, anxiety, and depression.
How Sickness Affects the Body and Mind:
Sickness can have a profound impact on both the body and mind. Physical sickness can cause a range of symptoms depending on the underlying condition, including fever, pain, weakness, nausea, and fatigue.

These symptoms can significantly affect the individual's ability to carry out daily activities and may require medical intervention.

Mental sickness, on the other hand, can manifest as emotional or behavioral changes such as irritability, anxiety, depression, or confusion.

It can affect the individual's ability to think, reason, or communicate effectively, and may require counseling or medication.

Both physical and mental sickness can also affect the individual's social and emotional well-being, leading to feelings of isolation, loneliness, and frustration. In severe cases, it can also lead to long-term disability or death.

The mind and sickness interact in complex ways. Our mental state can affect our physical health and vice versa. When we are under stress, anxious, or depressed, our immune system may become compromised, making us more susceptible to illnesses. Conversely, when we are physically ill, it can affect our mental state, leading to anxiety, depression, or other mental health issues. The mind can also affect how we perceive and experience sickness. Our thoughts and beliefs about illness can influence our immune response, pain tolerance, and recovery. For example, if we believe that we have a strong immune system and will recover quickly, it can help us feel more positive and hopeful, which can, in turn, support our physical healing.

On the other hand, negative thoughts and beliefs about illness, such as the belief that it is incurable or will lead to a significant loss, can lead to feelings of hopelessness and despair, which can negatively impact our physical recovery.

In addition, our mental state can also affect our behavior and lifestyle choices, which can have an impact on our physical health. For instance, stress and anxiety may lead to unhealthy coping mechanisms, such as smoking, drinking, or overeating, which can increase the risk of developing chronic illnesses.

Furthermore, the way we think and feel about sickness can also influence our adherence to treatment and our overall recovery. For instance, individuals who have positive beliefs and attitudes towards medical treatments and adhere to their medication regimens are more likely to achieve better health outcomes than those who do not.

On the other hand, negative beliefs and attitudes towards treatment, such as skepticism or mistrust of medical professionals, can lead to treatment non-adherence, which can undermine the effectiveness of medical interventions and prolong recovery.

In addition, the mind can also play a role in the development and exacerbation of certain illnesses, such as chronic pain or functional disorders.

Psychological factors such as stress, anxiety, and depression can contribute to the development and persistence of these conditions, leading to a vicious cycle of physical symptoms and mental distress.

Therefore, it is crucial to address the mental and emotional aspects of sickness to support our overall health and well-being.

This can include seeking appropriate medical care, managing stress and anxiety, and engaging in healthy coping mechanisms such as exercise, relaxation techniques, or therapy.

In conclusion, the interaction between the mind and sickness is complex and multi-faceted. Addressing the mental and emotional aspects of sickness is crucial to support our overall health and well-being, improve treatment adherence, and promote better health outcomes.

Chapter 13: The Physiology of Sickness

How the mind can influence the immune system:

The immune system is a complex network of cells, tissues, and organs that work together to protect the body against infections, diseases, and other harmful agents. The immune system is essential for maintaining overall health and well-being, and any dysfunction or impairment in its function can lead to the development of illnesses.

The immune system comprises various types of cells, such as white blood cells, antibodies, and cytokines, which work together to detect and destroy harmful agents, such as viruses, bacteria, and cancer cells. The immune system can also recognize and remember these agents to provide immunity against future infections.

The Effects of Stress on the Immune System:

Stress can have a significant impact on the immune system, particularly on the function of white blood cells. Chronic stress can suppress the immune response, leading to increased susceptibility to infections and diseases. Stress can also affect the production of cytokines, which are essential for regulating immune responses. Prolonged stress can lead to an overproduction of cytokines, causing inflammation and tissue damage.

Moreover, stress can also affect the production of antibodies, which are essential for providing immunity against infections. Chronic stress can lead to a decrease in the production of antibodies, leading to increased susceptibility to infections.

How Our Minds deal with our Immune System:

The mind can influence the immune system in various ways. For example, positive emotions such as happiness, joy, and love can stimulate the immune system, leading to increased production of antibodies and other immune cells.

On the other hand, negative emotions such as stress, anxiety, and depression can suppress the immune system, leading to decreased production of antibodies and increased susceptibility to infections.

The mind can also influence the immune system through various mechanisms such as the placebo effect. The placebo effect refers to the phenomenon where a person experiences a perceived improvement in symptoms, even though they received a non-active substance or treatment.

The placebo effect is believed to work by activating the body's natural healing mechanisms, including the immune system.

The placebo effect is often used in clinical trials to control for the effects of the mind on the immune system and other bodily processes.

There are various ways to support and boost the immune system. One way is to practice healthy lifestyle habits such as regular exercise, healthy diet, adequate sleep, and stress management techniques such as meditation, yoga, or deep breathing exercises.

These practices can help reduce stress and inflammation and boost the production of immune cells and antibodies.

Moreover, maintaining positive emotions and beliefs can also support immune function.

For instance, cultivating positive emotions such as gratitude, optimism, and resilience can help reduce stress and boost immune function.

Additionally, seeking social support and maintaining healthy relationships can also support immune function. Social support can provide a sense of comfort, safety, and belongingness, which can reduce stress and promote emotional well-being, leading to better immune function.

Furthermore, seeking appropriate medical care and adhering to prescribed treatments can also support immune function. This includes receiving vaccinations, taking prescribed medications as directed, and managing underlying medical conditions that can compromise immune function.

In conclusion, the immune system is essential for maintaining overall health and well-being, and any dysfunction or impairment in its function can lead to the development of illnesses. Stress can have a significant impact on the immune system, suppressing its function and increasing susceptibility to infections and diseases.

The mind can influence the immune system through various mechanisms, highlighting the importance of addressing mental and emotional factors in maintaining optimal immune function.

Chapter 14: Mind-Body Techniques for Healing

Mind-body techniques refer to a range of practices that aim to enhance the connection between the mind and body to promote healing, reduce stress, and improve overall well-being. These techniques recognize that the mind and body are interconnected and that emotional and mental states can influence physical health.

How Mind-Body Techniques Can Promote Healing:

Mind-body techniques can promote healing by reducing stress and promoting relaxation, which can lead to a decrease in inflammation and improve immune function. Additionally, mind-body techniques can help improve mood and emotional well-being, leading to an improvement in overall physical health.

Moreover, mind-body techniques can help individuals gain a sense of control and empowerment over their health and well-being. By practicing mind-body techniques, individuals can develop greater self-awareness and self-regulation skills, which can help them cope with physical and emotional challenges.

Techniques for Practicing Mind-Body Techniques:

There are various mind-body techniques that individuals can practice to promote healing and improve overall well-being. Here are some examples:

1.Meditation: Meditation involves the practice of focusing one's attention on a particular object or thought to promote relaxation, reduce stress, and improve emotional well-being.

2.Yoga: Yoga is a mind-body practice that combines physical postures, breathing techniques, and meditation to promote relaxation, reduce stress, and improve overall physical and emotional well-being.

3.Tai Chi: Tai Chi is an ancient Chinese practice that involves slow, graceful movements combined with deep breathing to promote relaxation, reduce stress, and improve physical and emotional well-being.

4.Guided Imagery: Guided imagery involves the practice of creating vivid mental images to promote relaxation, reduce stress, and improve overall well-being.

5.Biofeedback: Biofeedback involves the use of technology to monitor and provide feedback on physiological responses such as heart rate, muscle tension, and brain waves to help individuals learn to regulate these responses and reduce stress.

6.Progressive Muscle Relaxation: Progressive Muscle Relaxation (PMR) involves tensing and then relaxing various muscle groups to promote relaxation, reduce stress, and improve overall physical and emotional well-being.

7.Deep Breathing Exercises: Deep breathing exercises involve focusing on slow, deep breaths to promote relaxation, reduce stress, and improve overall physical and emotional well-being.

8.Mindfulness: Mindfulness involves the practice of being present in the moment and non-judgmentally observing one's thoughts, feelings, and bodily sensations to promote relaxation, reduce stress, and improve overall well-being.

9.Acupuncture: Acupuncture involves the insertion of thin needles into specific points on the body to promote relaxation, reduce pain, and improve overall physical and emotional well-being.

10.Massage: Massage involves the manipulation of soft tissues to promote relaxation, reduce stress, and improve overall physical and emotional well-being.

In conclusion, mind-body techniques can promote healing by enhancing the connection between the mind and body, reducing stress, and improving overall physical and emotional well-being. Practicing mind-body techniques such as meditation, yoga, Tai Chi, guided imagery, and biofeedback can help individuals develop greater self-awareness and self-regulation skills to support their health and well-being.

Chapter 15: Maintaining Our Mental health while Coping with Loss and Grief

Losing someone or something that is important to us can be a devastating experience that can impact our mental health. Grief is a natural response to loss, but it can also cause intense emotional pain, sadness, and other negative emotions that can be difficult to manage. Coping with grief and maintaining our mental health during this time is crucial to our overall well-being.

Here are some tips for maintaining your mental health while coping with loss and grief:

Acknowledge your feelings: It is essential to recognize and accept your feelings of sadness, anger, guilt, or any other emotions that come up during this time. Suppressing these feelings can lead to further emotional distress and may impact your mental health negatively.
Seek support: It is important to seek help from family, friends, or a support group to help you through your grieving process. Talking to someone who has experienced a similar loss can be comforting and helpful in understanding and processing your emotions. Professional counseling can also provide additional support if needed.

Take care of yourself: Take time to care for yourself physically, emotionally, and mentally. Get enough sleep, eat well, exercise, and engage in activities that you enjoy. Taking care of yourself can help you manage stress and improve your mood.

Accept that grief is a process: Grieving is a natural process that takes time. It is essential to be patient with yourself and allow yourself to feel your emotions and grieve at your own pace.

Practice mindfulness: Mindfulness techniques such as meditation or deep breathing can help reduce stress, calm your mind, and improve your overall mental health.

Be gentle with yourself: It is essential to be kind and compassionate to yourself during this time. Remember that grieving is a difficult process and that it is okay to take the time you need to heal.

Create new rituals: Creating new rituals or traditions can help honor your loved one's memory and create a sense of connection to them. This can be as simple as lighting a candle or planting a tree in their memory.

Find ways to express yourself: Finding a way to express your emotions and feelings can be helpful in processing your grief. You can write in a journal, create art, or talk to a trusted friend or family member.

Finding a healthy outlet to express your emotions can help you manage your feelings and reduce stress.

Keep a routine: Maintaining a routine can provide structure and stability during a time when everything else may feel out of control. This can include a regular sleep schedule, mealtimes, and daily activities. Having a routine can help you feel more grounded and provide a sense of normalcy.

Practice gratitude: Even in times of grief, there are things to be grateful for. Practicing gratitude can help shift your focus to the positive aspects of your life, even if they may seem small. You can keep a gratitude journal or simply take a few minutes each day to reflect on what you are thankful for.

It is important to remember that grief is a unique experience for everyone, and there is no right or wrong way to grieve. Be patient with yourself and allow yourself to feel your emotions. With time and support, you can heal and move forward while still cherishing the memories of your loved one.

In conclusion, coping with loss and grief is a challenging process that can impact our mental health. Taking care of ourselves, seeking support, and allowing ourselves to feel our emotions are essential steps in maintaining our mental health during this difficult time. Remember, grief is a natural process, and with time, healing is possible.

Chapter 16: Overcoming Negative Thoughts

Negative thoughts can have a profound impact on our minds and bodies, and can lead to a range of physical and mental health problems. In this chapter, we will explore the effects of negative thoughts on the mind and body, as well as techniques for overcoming them and cultivating positive thinking.

The Effects of Negative Thoughts on the Mind and Body

Negative thoughts can cause stress, anxiety, and depression, which can have a range of effects on our minds and bodies. Stress is a natural response to challenging situations, and in small doses, it can be beneficial. However, when we experience chronic stress, our bodies can become overwhelmed, leading to a range of physical symptoms, including headaches, muscle tension, and fatigue.

Chronic stress has also been linked to a range of health problems, including high blood pressure, heart disease, and obesity. When we are stressed, our bodies release stress hormones like cortisol and adrenaline. These hormones can increase blood pressure and heart rate, and cause inflammation in the body, which can contribute to the development of chronic diseases.

Cultivating positive thinking is an important part of overcoming negative thoughts. Here are some strategies for developing a more positive mindset:

Practice self-compassion: Treat yourself with kindness and understanding, even when things don't go as planned. Recognize that everyone makes mistakes, and that failure is an opportunity for growth.

Focus on strengths: Identify your strengths and focus on developing them. By focusing on your strengths, you can develop a greater sense of self-efficacy and confidence.

Surround yourself with positive people: Spending time with positive people can help you develop a more positive outlook on life. Positive people can inspire and motivate you, and provide you with support when you need it.

Engage in positive self-talk: Monitor your self-talk and replace negative thoughts with positive ones. For example, instead of saying "I'm not good enough," say "I'm doing my best and that's enough."

Set achievable goals: Setting goals can help you focus your energy and develop a sense of purpose. Make sure your goals are achievable and break them down into smaller steps to make them more manageable.

Negative thoughts can also affect our mental health. When we experience negative thoughts on a regular basis, we are more likely to develop anxiety and depression. These conditions can have a significant impact on our lives, making it difficult to enjoy daily activities and maintain healthy relationships.

Techniques for Overcoming Negative Thoughts

Fortunately, there are many techniques for overcoming negative thoughts. One of the most effective techniques is cognitive-behavioral therapy (as I mentioned earlier) or CBT which is a popular type of therapy that helps individuals identify and change negative thought patterns. It involves working with a therapist to develop new ways of thinking and behaving that are more positive and adaptive.

CBT is based on the idea that negative thoughts are learned behaviors that can be unlearned. By identifying and challenging negative thoughts, individuals can develop new ways of thinking that are more positive and adaptive. CBT also involves developing new behaviors that support positive thinking, such as engaging in activities that bring joy and fulfillment.

Another technique for overcoming negative thoughts (which I also mentioned earlier) is mindful meditation. Mindful meditation involves focusing on the present moment without judgment. By practicing mindfulness, individuals can learn to observe their thoughts without becoming attached to them. This can help them let go of negative thoughts and develop a more positive mindset.

Research has shown that mindfulness meditation can have a range of benefits, including reducing stress and anxiety, improving mood, and enhancing cognitive function. Mindfulness meditation can also help individuals develop a greater sense of self-awareness, which can lead to greater emotional regulation and resilience.

Other techniques for overcoming negative thoughts include:

Journaling: Writing down negative thoughts can help individuals identify patterns and develop new ways of thinking.

Once again, Gratitude practice: Focusing on the positive aspects of life can help shift attention away from negative thoughts. Practicing gratitude can also help individuals develop a greater sense of well-being and happiness.

Physical activity: Exercise can release endorphins, which can improve mood and reduce stress. Regular exercise can also help individuals develop a greater sense of self-efficacy and confidence.

How to Cultivate Positive Thinking:

Practice mindfulness: As mentioned earlier, practicing mindfulness can help you let go of negative thoughts and develop a more positive mindset. Try incorporating mindfulness into your daily routine by practicing meditation, yoga, or simply taking a few moments to focus on your breath. Engage in activities that bring you joy: Doing things you enjoy can boost your mood and help you develop a greater sense of fulfillment. Make time for activities that bring you joy, whether it's reading a book, listening to music, or spending time with loved ones.

Conclusion:

Negative thoughts can have a significant impact on our lives, both mentally and physically. However, there are many techniques for overcoming negative thoughts and developing a more positive mindset. Cognitive-behavioral therapy, mindfulness meditation, journaling, gratitude practice, and physical activity are just a few of the strategies that can help you overcome negative thinking patterns. By cultivating positive thinking and engaging in activities that bring you joy, you can improve your mental and physical health and live a more fulfilling life.

Chapter 17: Snooze or Lose: Sleep and its Impact on Mental Health

We've all been there - tossing and turning in bed, counting sheep, and praying for the sweet relief of sleep. But did you know that lack of sleep can have a significant impact on your mental health? In this chapter, we'll explore the importance of sleep and its impact on mental health, and offer some tips for getting a better night's rest. So put on your pajamas, fluff up your pillows, and let's dive in!

The Importance of Sleep

Sleep is essential for our physical and mental well-being. It allows our bodies to rest and repair, and our brains to process information and emotions. Without adequate sleep, we can experience a range of physical and mental health problems.

For example, lack of sleep can lead to fatigue, irritability, and difficulty concentrating. It can also weaken our immune system, making us more susceptible to illness. In the long term, chronic sleep deprivation has been linked to a range of health problems, including obesity, diabetes, and heart disease.

But perhaps the most significant impact of sleep deprivation is on our mental health. Lack of sleep can lead to anxiety, depression, and other mood disorders. It can also exacerbate symptoms of existing mental health conditions.

The Link Between Sleep and Mental Health:

There are many ways in which sleep can impact our mental health. For one, sleep deprivation can interfere with the brain's ability to regulate emotions. This can lead to mood swings, irritability, and difficulty managing stress.

Sleep deprivation can also lead to cognitive impairments, such as difficulty concentrating, poor memory, and decreased productivity. These cognitive impairments can make it difficult to perform well at work or school, and can contribute to feelings of anxiety and stress.

In addition, sleep deprivation can impact our social and emotional functioning. When we're sleep-deprived, we may be more likely to withdraw from social interactions and feel less connected to others. This can contribute to feelings of loneliness and depression.

Tips for Getting a Better Night's Rest:

Now that we've established the importance of sleep for mental health, let's discuss some tips for getting a better night's rest. Here are some strategies you can try:

Stick to a sleep schedule: Try to go to bed and wake up at the same time every day, even on weekends. This can help regulate your body's sleep-wake cycle and improve the quality of your sleep.

Create a relaxing bedtime routine: Establish a relaxing bedtime routine to signal to your body that it's time to wind down. This could include taking a warm bath, reading a book, or practicing relaxation techniques like deep breathing.

Create a sleep-conducive environment: Make sure your bedroom is cool, quiet, and dark. Use comfortable bedding and pillows to create a comfortable sleep environment. Limit caffeine and alcohol intake: Avoid consuming caffeine and alcohol in the hours leading up to bedtime. Both substances can interfere with your ability to fall and stay asleep.
Get regular exercise: Regular exercise can improve sleep quality and duration.

Aim for at least 30 minutes of moderate-intensity exercise per day, but make sure to finish your workout at least a few hours before bedtime.

Limit screen time before bed: Exposure to the blue light emitted by electronic devices can interfere with your body's production of melatonin, a hormone that regulates sleep. Try to limit your exposure to screens in the hours leading up to bedtime.

Sleep is essential for our physical and mental well-being. Lack of sleep can lead to a range of health problems, including anxiety, depression, and other mood disorders. However, by adopting some healthy sleep habits, you can improve the quality and duration of your sleep and support your mental health. So put on those comfy pajamas, fluff up those pillows, and get ready for some sweet dreams!

Don't force sleep: Trying too hard to fall asleep can actually make it harder to do so. If you're struggling to fall asleep, try getting out of bed and doing something relaxing, like reading a book or practicing a mindfulness exercise.

Seek help if needed: If you're struggling with chronic sleep problems or experiencing symptoms of a sleep disorder, it's important to seek help from a healthcare professional.

They can help you identify the underlying causes of your sleep problems and recommend appropriate treatments.

Humor is a great way to reduce stress and improve our mood, and it can also help us approach serious topics like sleep and mental health with a more lighthearted perspective. So, in the spirit of humor, here are some bonus tips for getting a good night's sleep:

Invest in a high-quality mattress and pillows, because nothing says "sweet dreams" like sinking into a cloud of fluffiness.

Try sleeping with a weighted blanket, because who needs a significant other when you can snuggle with a 25-pound piece of fabric?
Wear socks to bed, because nothing says "sexy" like a pair of fuzzy socks and a flannel nightgown.
And finally, if all else fails, count sheep...or unicorns, or llamas, or whatever animal brings you joy.
In all seriousness, sleep is a vital component of our overall health and well-being. By prioritizing sleep and adopting healthy sleep habits, we can improve our mental health and live happier, more fulfilling lives. So go ahead and embrace your inner sloth, and remember: snooze or lose!

Chapter 18. The Mind-Body Connection in Chronic Pain:

Chronic pain is a complex phenomenon that affects millions of people around the world. It can be caused by a variety of conditions, including arthritis, fibromyalgia, migraines, and back pain, among others. While chronic pain is often thought of as a physical problem, recent research has shown that it is also strongly influenced by psychological factors. This connection between the mind and body is referred to as the mind-body connection.

The mind-body connection is based on the idea that the mind and body are not separate entities, but are interconnected and influence each other. This means that the way we think, feel, and behave can have a significant impact on our physical health, including the experience of chronic pain. Studies have shown that people who experience chronic pain often have higher levels of stress, anxiety, and depression, which can exacerbate their physical symptoms.

One of the key ways that thoughts and emotions can affect physical symptoms is through the stress response. When we experience stress, our body releases hormones such as cortisol and adrenaline, which can increase inflammation and cause pain. In addition, stress can lead to muscle tension and poor posture, which can contribute to the development of chronic pain.

Another way that thoughts and emotions can affect chronic pain is through the placebo effect. The placebo effect is a well-known phenomenon in which people experience a reduction in symptoms after receiving a treatment that is inactive or has no therapeutic effect. While the placebo effect is often dismissed as a trick of the mind, research has shown that it can be a powerful tool for reducing pain and improving overall health.

Mind-body interventions such as cognitive-behavioral therapy, mindfulness-based stress reduction, and meditation have been shown to be effective in reducing chronic pain. These interventions work by helping people to identify and change negative thought patterns, manage stress and anxiety, and develop more positive coping strategies. They also encourage people to become more mindful of their physical sensations, which can help them to better understand and manage their pain.

In addition to mind-body interventions, lifestyle factors such as diet and exercise can also play a role in the mind-body connection. Eating a healthy diet and engaging in regular physical activity can help to reduce inflammation and improve overall health, which can in turn reduce the experience of chronic pain.

Overall, the mind-body connection in chronic pain is a complex and multifaceted phenomenon that is influenced by a variety of factors. By understanding the connection between our thoughts, emotions, and physical symptoms, we can develop more effective strategies for managing chronic pain and improving our overall health and well-being.

One important aspect of the mind-body connection in chronic pain is the role of negative emotions such as fear, anger, and depression. These emotions can amplify the experience of pain, making it feel more intense and more difficult to manage. For example, people with chronic pain may develop a fear of movement or exercise due to the belief that it will worsen their pain. This fear can lead to decreased physical activity and increased pain, creating a cycle of avoidance and increased suffering.

On the other hand, positive emotions such as hope, gratitude, and joy can help to reduce pain and improve overall well-being. Research has shown that cultivating a sense of gratitude can help to reduce stress and improve mood, which can in turn reduce the experience of pain. Similarly, engaging in activities that bring joy and pleasure can help to distract from pain and improve overall quality of life.

Another important factor in the mind-body connection is the role of social support. Chronic pain can be a isolating and lonely experience, but having a supportive network of friends, family, and healthcare providers can help to reduce the emotional burden and improve overall coping. Support groups and peer-to-peer programs can also provide a sense of community and belonging, which can be especially helpful for people with chronic pain.

Finally, it's important to recognize that the mind-body connection is not a one-way street. While negative thoughts and emotions can worsen
chronic pain, chronic pain can also lead to negative thoughts and emotions. For example, feeling trapped in a cycle of pain and disability can lead to feelings of hopelessness and despair. Recognizing and addressing these negative emotions is an important part of managing chronic pain and improving overall well-being.

Overall, the mind-body connection in chronic pain is a complex and multifaceted phenomenon that requires a holistic approach to management. By recognizing the role of thoughts, emotions, and social support, people with chronic pain can develop effective strategies for reducing pain and improving our quality of life.